aging
well

aging well

30 Lessons for Making the Most of Your Later Years

Janice Walton, PhD

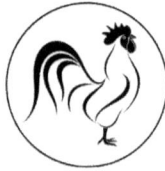

Rooster Press

P.O. Box 1654

Pleasanton, CA 94566

www.roosterpress.com

ISBN: 978-1-949378-05-4

First printing, 2020.

Printed by Kindle Direct Publishing in the United States of America.

Copyediting by Geri Walton

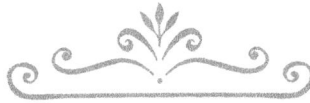

Contents

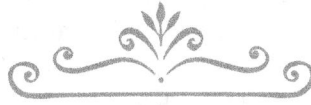

Introduction

Oh, oh!!! Whether you think of it as retirement, getting old, or transitioning to a new chapter in life, most of us reach a pivotal point when we realize life is entering its later stages. Yet, as people live longer, they need to find engaging, stimulating ways to continue to grow personally, and many have no idea what to do in their so-called golden years. So, a question to consider is "how do you want to spend the rest of your life—aging optimally or going slowly downhill until death? *Aging optimally* means to be the person you want to be despite life's stresses.

Aging optimally can be challenging these days due to the myths and misinformation that abound and the circumstances that inevitably arise. It is a choice, you know! You can develop qualities that can help you make the journey much more rewarding.

At the time of this book, my husband and I were 81 years of age. We met when we were 12 and had been married for 61 years. We were born and raised in Ohio, moved to California, and lived in the state of Washington for several years before returning to California, family, and the sun. We had two children with two grandsons. You could think of me as a rebel. I never wanted to be like everyone else or to be the old person portrayed on television: A person who makes poor decisions, is easily victimized, and is waiting for ailments to overtake them until they die. That was not going to be my life story. With such a mindset, I went to work for a police department when I was 50, earned a PhD in Psychology when I was 60, and moved out of state when I was 70. Now I am committed to exploring how best to age optimally. My husband and I eat nutritiously, exercise regularly, and take no prescription drugs. We both worked full time until two years ago. While we are basically healthy, we do experience aches and pains. In addition, I recently had cataract surgery. My husband has also experienced increased memory loss after surgery; perhaps, due to the medications and anesthesia given during his hospital stay. While the surgery may have been necessary, our lives have changed dramatically since then.

This booklet chronicles my quest to age optimally and is based on my experience. To help you benefit from what I have learned, I offer thirty mini-lessons that include insights, ideas, and goals for you to consider and achieve if you wish to age optimally as well. To help you understand the lessons, here is a brief overview:

- **Lesson 1**: Discusses myths and misinformation regarding older adults.

- **Lessons 2 to 4:** Provides three informal assessment tools that can help you: a) evaluate your satisfaction with life, b) identify what can and can't be accomplished realistically, and c) establish a goal for moving forward.

- **Lessons 5 to 20:** Describes helpful qualities for aging optimally, qualities that can be learned.

- **Lessons 21 to 30**: Identifies stressors and situations that may challenge your goal and offers tools for managing those challenges.

Creating change in your life doesn't have to happen slowly, it can occur quickly. If you read this book and incorporate a new lesson each day, you may find yourself in a much better position in just a few short weeks and you, too, can age optimally. Are you ready? Let's begin!

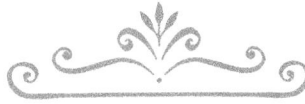

Lesson 1

Myths and Misinformation

Society's attitude about age is embedded in the term *ageism*. Ageism occurs when an older person is treated unfairly. Ageism can occur when the person loses a job, is refused a new credit card, receives poor service in a shop or less than quality care from a doctor, or is denied membership to a club just because of his or her age.

Ageism extends to the way older people are represented in the media and causes an impact on public attitudes, as well. For some reason, older adults, aren't portrayed as wise, weathered or intelligent; rather they are portrayed as sweet, naïve, and vulnerable. News stories featuring them as crime victims are a natural extension of this narrative. Daily headlines such as the following often appear: "Elderly Savannah woman scammed out of her life savings", "Police hunt driver who hit elderly man in wheelchair then fled" and "Elderly man missing in Torrington." Such headlines show older people in need of protection and care. This portrayal makes it easier for their opinions, concerns, and contributions to be discounted. A University of Southern California study also noted:[1]

> *"If you watch TV, you're likely to hear ageist language, see worn-out stereotypes, and wonder why older characters lead such one-dimensional lives. That's if older adults*

---

[1]   Lisa Esposito, *Ageism in Top TV Shows May Affect Seniors' Well-Being*, https://health.usnews.com/wellness/articles/2017-10-18/ageism-in-top-tv-shows-may-affect-seniors-well-being, 8/16/20.

> *even exist, much less speak, on your favorite shows.*
> *Seniors are underrepresented on screen, behind the*
> *camera and as TV writers and producers."*

This underlying attitude, inaccurate media portrayals, and a lack of adequate education on aging combine to produce a myriad of myths and misinformation. While there are many myths, popular ones are that old people have "old ways" of thinking, elderly people are less adaptable to change and less adventurous, and "old people'" are crabby, depressed, and lonely. People are peppered with assumptions about aging, many of which are just not true. Furthermore, older adults often internalize the low expectations conveyed in these portrayals, which in turn creates the foundation for a self-fulfilling prophecy.

Ironically, the age at which a person is considered elderly depends on what you read. The Social Security Administration says elderly is 65+. They determine who is eligible for benefits accordingly. The **Merriam Webster dictionary** defines elderly as being past middle age. To me, the word has more to do with a person's mindset and ability to function rather than on a number.

Anne Tergesen writer for the *Wall Street Journal* covering retirement offers words of hope.[2] She says everyone believes that as we age, our minds and bodies decline, life becomes less satisfying and enjoyable, and we become less productive at work. The hope Ms Tergesen offers is that everyone it seems is wrong. There are many older adults who agree. Think about 85-year old Dianne Feinstein the senator from California, or 88-year-old Warren Buffet the highly regarded CEO of Berkshire Hathaway, or 96-year old Betty White, the actress, activist, and comedian to name a few.

---

[2]   Anne Tergeson, (video) *Why Everything You Think About Aging May Be Wrong*, https://www.wsj.com/articles/why-everything-you-think-about-aging-may-be-wrong-1417408057 8/16/20.

PRACTICE

To practice, take a minute to consider myths and misinformation about aging that may influence your thinking and decisions. Make a list of them. Now, ask yourself whether they are helpful or harmful. Did you identify any that you want to reconsider?

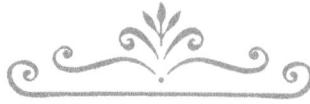

Lesson 2

Personal House Cleaning

So, here you are at Lesson 2! Despite the prevailing mindset or misinformation, you have chosen to age optimally. You want to succeed despite life's challenges and stresses. This second lesson will help you assess how happy you are with life, identify helpful qualities you possess, and determine challenges and stresses that may be occurring. To accomplish this, begin by completing a personal house cleaning assessment regarding things you like about your life, things you want to change in your life, your strengths and weaknesses, and challenges and opportunities, you face.

PRACTICE

To conduct your house cleaning, ask yourself the following eight questions

1. What bothers you?
2. What "shoulds" and frustrations nag you?
3. What daily habits support you and your goals?
4. What saps your energy?
5. What drains you?
6. What about relationships?
7. What goals inspire you?
8. What are your strengths?

When I completed the house cleaning assessment, three goals were clear: I want to age optimally, spend time with family, and share my ideas with others. It's your turn to complete the assessment. Then, ask yourself what you learned and what you want to do about it.

Lesson 3

Your New Normal

In the previous lessons, you identified myths and misinformation that can adversely affect your goal to age optimally, and you conducted a personal house cleaning. The next step is determining what normal is for you now. As the past president of a Canadian Seniors Association said:[3]

> *"I don't know what would be considered normal aging. What's normal for a 45-year-old? What's normal for an 80-year-old? Those are really irrelevant terms as far as I'm concerned."*

As she suggested there really is no such thing as normal aging. Each person is unique and changes over time. However, the truth is that your energy level, motivation, and dreams don't remain the same. So, an evaluation of your current strengths and weakness minus excuses, denial, and unwillingness to accept what is true seems wise.

Such an evaluation might include questions such as: What can I actually accomplish in a day? What are my excuses for not doing what I want and are they legitimate? Do I have a purpose for the future and what is it? Am I kidding myself about what I can and can't do?

---

[3] University of Alberta, *Defining the new normal in aging*, https://www.sciencedaily.com/releases/2013/02/130227113058.htm, 8/16/20.

PRACTICE

Now take a few minutes to analyze your life. After answering these or similar questions, you can develop a life plan based on what is now normal for you. This plan, which may change in a few months, should focus on what you can do, provide solutions for difficult situations, and include options.

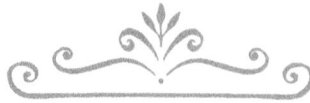

Lesson 4

Achieving a Goal

Based on your personal housecleaning and your new normal, the final step is to create a goal for aging optimally. You can use the following process (adapted *from an iNLP Center strategy*) to clearly define it. That is what 65-year-old Jennifer did. Jennifer is a single woman, who recently retired after working for a major company the past 35 years. She conducted a personal housecleaning, determined her new normal, and decided to develop a plan for the rest of her life.

The nine questions she asked herself and her responses are as follows:

1. What do you want?
   Jennifer: I want to develop a plan to be the best I can despite my circumstances; to age optimally.
2. How will you know when you have reached the goal? What do you want to happen and with whom?
   Jennifer: I will have a plan for responding to life situations with confidence and resilience. I want to remain actively engaged in all areas of my life.
3. What will you hear, see, and feel as you achieve this goal?
   Jennifer: I'll hear myself speaking optimistically, I'll see myself making healthy choices, and I'll feel confident with my future plan.
4. Why is your goal relevant?
   Jennifer: I want to have a plan for contributing to life rather than depending on others.

5. What stops you from pursuing your goal wholeheartedly?
    Jennifer: I have many excuses and am easily discouraged.
6. What personal resources can you use to achieve this goal?
    Jennifer: I am healthy, willing, and
    committed to personal development.
7. What additional resources do you need to achieve your
    goal?
    Jennifer: I need patience and persistence to develop
    the plan, as well as, motivation to implement it.
8. How can your goal affect important people in your life?
    What gets in the way?
    Jennifer: My family is thrilled with my plan. They
    don't have to worry about taking care of me. However,
    staying on track is difficult. I lose focus, at times.
9. What daily actions must you take to achieve your goal?
    What is the first step?
    Jennifer: I must focus on what I can do and solutions,
    and create a plan that works for me. The first step
    is to examine my beliefs and perceptions.

Jennifer included what she learned from completing the exercise as she developed her plan. When she took the first step of examining her beliefs and perceptions, she found several that were holding her back.

PRACTICE

You, too, can examine any goal just as Jennifer did. Do so by asking yourself the same or similar questions. Maybe you will learn important information as she did.

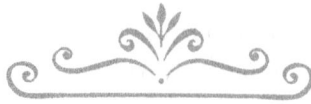

Lesson 5

Purpose

The literature on optimal aging says that having a life purpose and a healthy life-style are important. I have found other qualities are involved; so, let's briefly examine each of them.

Purpose is unique to everyone because what you identify as your path will likely be different from someone else's path. What's more, your purpose may shift and change in response to the changing priorities and fluctuations of life. You need to consider what adds satisfaction to your life. Determining your purpose and living a meaningful life may not be as difficult as it seems. For instance, my purpose is to age optimally and to be there for my family. You can identify your purpose by defining what is important to you, having the courage to express yourself, and focusing on what has meaning for you.

PRACTICE

Three questions to ask as you reflect on your life purpose are as follows:

1. Who am I?
2. Where do I belong?
3. When do I feel fulfilled?

You may finally have the time you were yearning for all those years when raising a family and working. What was it you wanted to do, but didn't get around to? If nothing comes to mind easily, don't worry. For some, discovering a new purpose takes time and soul-searching. So, don't be discouraged if you don't have an immediate answer. Begin by asking yourself the three questions above, and once you have identified a possible purpose see if that makes a difference in your thinking. However, remember, your purpose may change as situations change.

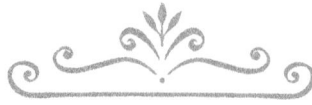

Lesson 6

A Healthy Lifestyle

Most of the literature focuses on the need for people to be physically healthy as they age. Physical health includes exercise, preventing and managing disease, and nutritious eating. The literature on optimal aging suggests that a healthy lifestyle also includes functional, cognitive, emotional, social, and spiritual wellness. Functional wellness focuses on living effectively.

- **Cognitive wellness** looks at brain health and the ability to find pleasure, meaning, purpose, and fulfillment in life.

- **Emotional wellness** reminds me of the term emotional intelligence (EQ). According to Howard Gardner, the Harvard theorist, "EQ is the level of your ability to understand other people, what motivates them and how to work cooperatively with them." Gardner named five important skills for implementing EQ: self-awareness, self-regulation, motivation, empathy, and social connectedness.

- **Social wellness** involves healthy, nurturing, and supportive relationships as well as fostering connections with those around you.

- **Spiritual wellness** is generally considered to be the search for meaning and purpose that leads a person to strive for a state of harmony with him or herself and others while working to balance inner needs with the demands of life. The path to spiritual wellness can involve meditation, mindfulness, prayer, and affirmations that support your connection to a higher power or belief system. This higher power can be thought of as the Universe, God, Spirit, or an Inner Guide.

PRACTICE

One way to evaluate your spiritual wellness is by asking these four questions

1. Do I make time for relaxation every day?
2. Do I make time for meditation and/or prayer?
3. Do my values guide my decisions and actions?
4. Am I able to accept the views of others? You might want to examine your lifestyle and ask yourself where you can improve.

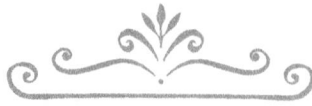

Lesson 7

Resilience

Now that you have completed lessons 1 through 6, your next question is probably "what qualities do I need to get started on my way to optimal aging?" The following lessons (7 through 20) identify factors that can be helpful. If these qualities are not something you currently possess, the good news is that they can be learned. Even though these qualities don't guarantee optimal aging, they can help make life more manageable.

The first factor we will discuss is resilience. Resilience is the ability to bounce back from difficult experiences. Resilience involves behaviors, thoughts, and actions that can be developed by anyone. Lyrics from an old Frank Sinatra song describe resilience well, "pick yourself up, dust yourself off, and start all over again."

Many studies suggest a primary factor in maintaining resilience is caring and supportive relationships. Additional factors include the capacity to make realistic plans and carry them out, a positive sense of self, confidence in one's identified strengths and abilities, skills in communication and problem solving, and an ability to manage strong feelings and impulses.

PRACTICE

Resilience is built when you do the 14 items listed below. So, select two or three and begin today to incorporate them into your life.

1. Disregard the belief that crises are insurmountable. You can't change the fact that highly stressful events happen, but you can change how you interpret them and respond.
2. Accept change as a part of living. That means certain goals may no longer be attainable because of circumstances.
3. Accept circumstances that can't be changed and focus on those that can. The serenity prayer seems to fit.

God, grant me the **serenity** to accept the things I cannot change, the **courage** to change the things I can, and the **wisdom** to know the difference.

CAMEN Designs

4. Ask yourself "What can I do today that helps me move in the direction I want to go?"
5. Take decisive action when you can.
6. Look for opportunities to self-discover.
7. Develop confidence in your ability to solve problems and to trust your instincts.
8. Even when facing painful situations, consider the stressful situation in a broader context and keep a long-term perspective.
9. Maintain a hopeful outlook. Visualize what you want, rather than worry about what you fear.
10. Take care of yourself by engaging in activities that are relaxing and enjoyable for you.

11. Keep a journal and meditate to help restore your hope.
12. Identify ways that are most likely to work for you.
13. Find others in similar situations who can be supportive.

Lesson 8

Resourcefulness

Resourcefulness is a beneficial factor in living an optimal life. It's one thing to have a good idea, but it can be much harder to find ways to execute your idea. Resourcefulness is the ability to think creatively, to generate ideas, to identify alternatives, and to visualize how something can be achieved even though there is nothing but a vision. The term "thinking outside the box comes to mind." Resourceful people tend to bend the rules, look for a common good, adapt and apply other experiences, have more than one plan, ask for what they need, and say yes to themselves more often. It's easy to have creative ideas, but ignoring them can be sabotaging.

PRACTICE

Think of a situation that you were unable to resolve and apply those guidelines to determine if you would have been happier with the results. Maybe, you didn't receive a rebate for a recent purchase even though you followed the procedures for requesting a rebate. To solve the issue, you contact the corporate offices and research getting help from a television hotline. During the conversation with the corporate offices, you explain what you need without apologizing and suggest that it would be in their best interest to send the rebate immediately. Otherwise, you will contact the hotline for help. Would that approach have been more effective for you? If not, what approach might help you solve the problem?

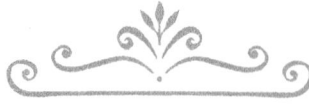

Lesson 9

Willingness

Willingness is defined as being disposed or inclined to be prepared, to act or be ready to act gladly, or to accept voluntarily or ungrudgingly. Maybe willingness can be thought of as the ability to adapt as circumstances change with a cheerful readiness. In the case of wanting to age optimally, willingness means committing to take important actions related to your goal. Willingness means feeling the anxieties, stressors, and fears, that may occur. When life asks whether you are willing to experience fear to move forward or to accept the new normal; then, your answer must be yes.

A major aspect of willingness is emotional resilience, which refers to one's ability to adapt to stressful situations and crises in a healthy way. Emotionally resilient people adapt to adversity without lasting difficulties whereas less emotionally resilient people have a harder time with stress and accepting life changes.

PRACTICE

Consider a situation where you embraced willingness. How did that change the outcome or did it make the situation any easier?

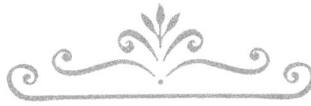

Lesson 10

Motivation

Motivation can be thought of as moving away from negative outcomes or moving toward positive ones. People who "move away" avoid difficulty but may not consider what they really want. People who "move toward" focus on what is pleasant and desirable but ignore potential problems and fail to prepare for them. How often have you forced yourself to do things you should do but don't want to do such as cleaning the garage? How easy is it for you to go to the gym when your friend invites you to go shopping? These activities require motivation to accomplish them. Motivating factors can include a good reason, a goal you want to achieve and a plan, flexibility, taking small steps, and learning from mistakes.

Motivation is a pulling force. It is something from the outside that compels you to act. People say that inspiration or desperation can be driving forces for change as well. However, inspiration is probably healthier than desperation because it has a greater chance of being connected to your purpose. You may be motivated to take classes and volunteer because friends say you "should," but if you are inspired to age optimally, you do those things because you want to be the best you can be for as long as possible. Being the best may include taking classes and volunteering.

Practice

Next time you have trouble completing a project, take the time to identify the motivating or inspiring factors that will help you move forward.

Lesson 11

A Positive Attitude

You may have heard that an important ingredient in aging is having a positive attitude. A positive attitude encompasses the range of life's experiences. It is truly a way of being and can be summarized in the following way:[4]

> *"It's believing in good times during bad times. It's feeling grateful for what you have instead of lamenting on what you lack. It's believing not simply that the positive outweighs the negative in life, but that we can create positive feelings and actions; that we have the power to make ourselves happy and content. From an aging perspective, it can also mean accepting limitations without surrendering to them."*

Another consideration is explanatory style. This refers to how people explain to themselves why they experience a certain event, whether positively or negatively, optimistically or pessimistically. There are three aspects to identifying your explanatory style. The first aspect is personal: an optimist tends to think "things happen" and the

---

[4] Chicago Tribune, *A positive mental attitude benefits health, longevity and quality of life,* https://www.chicagotribune.com/real-estate/chi-primetime-pma-022611-story.html , 8/16/20.

pessimist thinks "it is my fault." The second aspect is permanence. An optimist tends to define failure as transitory, "I didn't study enough" and the pessimist defines his failure as permanent, "I'm never good at tests." The final aspect is pervasive. An optimist tends to think "I have had dealings with mostly honest people" and the pessimist thinks "Everyone is out to get me."

PRACTICE

If your explanatory style is pessimistic, you may want to work on viewing circumstances in a more positive light. Take a moment to write down 10 things that are positive about your life now. How do you feel when you read this list?

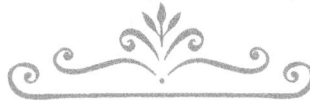

Lesson 12

Perception

Your explanatory style is impacted by your perceptions and beliefs. So, let's discuss perceptions first. Perceptions refer to how you make sense of the world around you. They are mental states or conditions that influence the way you see and understand things. While both states are influential, I think internal factors play a greater role than external ones in shaping a person's perceptions

Five influential internal factors are:

- Beliefs that influence perception. We are taught to believe only what we see. If you can't see it, then it's not real. In truth, it is believing is seeing.

- Expectations that influence how you perceive something. If you expect snakes to be scary, they will be.

- Your mindset, which may be impacted by explanatory style.

- Ignoring information that creates conflict or threatens you. You may not want to admit you gained 25 pounds over the last five years or that the weight you gained may be harmful to your health.

- Acknowledging new information but treating it as an exception. You might notice there is an increase in extreme weather, but see it as "a fluke" rather than a new pattern.

External factors are that bigger size attracts the attention of the perceiver, a loud sound, strong odor, or bright light is noticed more than a soft sound, weak odor or dim light, and a moving object draws more attention than a static one.

PRACTICE

Make a list of your perceptions about aging and ask yourself how well they serve you.

Lesson 13

Beliefs

Now let's briefly talk about beliefs. Tony Robbins, an American author, entrepreneur, philanthropist, motivational speaker, and life coach, once said:[5]

> *Human beings have the awesome ability to take any experience of their lives and create a meaning that disempowers them or one that can literally save their lives.*

Our beliefs are based on perceptions we accept as valid. However, just because we view things in a certain way doesn't mean they are really that way. Beliefs affect our actions, determine our quality of life, and serve us.

The power of belief was described in the book, *Pygmalion in the Classroom* (2003), by psychologist Robert Rosenthal. In a well-known study, a group of average intelligent school children were randomly divided into two equal groups. One group was assigned to a teacher who was told her students were "gifted." The other group was assigned to a teacher who was told her students were "slow learners." A year later the two groups were retested. Most of the "gifted" students scored higher than they had previously, while

---

[5] **Tony Robbins, Brainy Quote, https://www.brainyquote.com/quotes/ tony_robbins_147773, 8/16/20.**

most of the "slow" learners scored lower. The teachers' beliefs affected student performance.

PRACTICE

Think about the beliefs you hold. Do they move you toward your goals or do they create stress? An interesting experiment is to list five to ten beliefs you have and ask whether they serve you well. Do that now. If you find your beliefs don't serve you well, consider more empowering ones. You may be surprised how irrational some of those beliefs are and how new beliefs can change your life for the better.

As Tony Robbins said,[6]

> *"If you want to succeed, it would be wise for you to choose your beliefs carefully, rather than walking around like a piece of flypaper, picking up whichever belief sticks. An important thing to realize is that the potentials we tap, the results we get, are all part of a dynamic process that begins with belief."*

If you are not aware of your perceptions and beliefs and don't know they can be changed, you may be stuck in old ways of being and thinking. The exciting news is that you can change them. Just as you look at a photo from another angle, you can look at life differently. There are many options. If you change your perceptions and beliefs, you change your reality, and in turn, you change your life.

---

[6]   Tony Robbins. *Unlimited Power.*

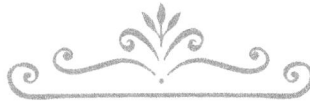

Lesson 14

Mindfulness

Two major ways to relieve stress are mindfulness and meditation. Mindfulness is the basic human practice of returning to the present moment, being aware of where you are and what you are doing, while not be overly reactive or overwhelmed by what's going on. When you focus on what you're directly experiencing using your senses, emotions, and mind, you are being mindful.

Mindfulness is available every minute, whether you are practicing meditation, pausing, or breathing when the phone rings instead of rushing to answer it. Mindfulness helps you put space between yourself and your reactions and breaks down habitual responses.

Basic strategies for being mindful include setting aside a time and space, and observing your body sensations, feelings, or thoughts. The goal of mindfulness is to pay attention to the present moment without judgment, letting your judgments pass by like clouds floating in the sky.

Mindfulness can help relieve stress, treat heart disease, lower blood pressure, reduce chronic pain, improve sleep, and alleviate gastrointestinal difficulties. By focusing on the here and now, you are less likely to get caught up in worries about the future or regrets over the past, less preoccupied with concerns regarding success and self-esteem, and better able to form deep connections with others. In recent years, therapists have turned to mindfulness meditation in the treatment of problems such as depression, substance abuse, eating disorders, and couples' conflicts.

PRACTICE

Try practicing mindfulness for a few days, you may find it very helpful.

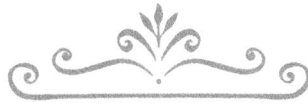

Lesson 15

Meditation

Like mindfulness, meditation helps you manage stress. The two practices complement each other, and very often overlap. At the same time, each has its own specific definition and purpose. As mentioned, mindfulness is the act of focusing on being in the present. An example would be to totally focus on drinking a cup of hot tea, taking in its scent and taste, feeling its warmth, and removing overpowering emotions from the mind. Meditation is a term that encompasses the practice of reaching ultimate consciousness and concentration, to acknowledge the mind and, in a way, self-regulate it. It can involve numerous techniques or practices to reach this heightened level of consciousness — including compassion, love, patience, and of course, mindfulness. So, mindfulness is a type of meditation, like yoga and breathing.

PRACTICE

One way to meditate is to sit or lie comfortably, close your eyes, breathe naturally, and focus your attention on your breath and on how the body moves with each inhalation and exhalation. You can also focus on a word or a sound. For example, when breathing in repeat the word "peace" and when breathing out repeat the word "stress." I am learning to use mindfulness and it does make a difference. The process takes me away from the useless chatter of everyday life that goes on in my mind and relieves stress.

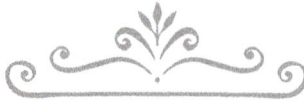

Lesson 16

Gratitude

Gratitude is an emotion expressing appreciation for what one has as opposed to what one **wants** or **needs**. A half-hearted "thanks" isn't enough: Deep gratitude comes from within and is felt in a meaningful way. The benefits of gratitude are expressed in the diagram below,[7] and they are important in your desire to age optimally.

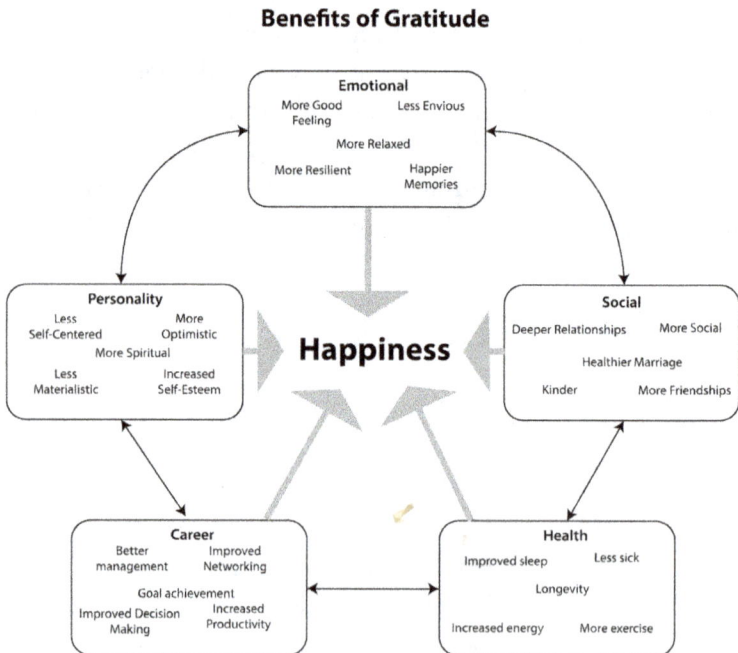

Benefits of Gratitude

Emotional
More Good Feeling   Less Envious
More Relaxed
More Resilient   Happier Memories

Personality
Less Self-Centered   More Optimistic
More Spiritual
Less Materialistic   Increased Self-Esteem

Happiness

Social
Deeper Relationships   More Social
Healthier Marriage
Kinder   More Friendships

Career
Better management   Improved Networking
Goal achievement
Improved Decision Making   Increased Productivity

Health
Improved sleep   Less sick
Longevity
Increased energy   More exercise

---

7   http://happierhuman.com/benefits-of-gratitude/

PRACTICE

How does someone cultivate gratitude? Here are seven options to consider:

1. Be amazed at the goodness you typically take for granted.
2. Maintain a gratitude journal or diary of things for which you are grateful. Review it regularly.
3. Give a compliment daily.
4. When the situation is bad, ask yourself what you can learn and what you can be grateful for.
5. Vow not to complain, criticize or gossip for a week.
6. Express your gratitude out loud.
7. Look for things to be grateful for in your everyday life.

There are many things to be grateful for even if you have problems; so, make a gratitude list or diary. When life seems difficult, review the list to remind yourself of the good in your life. Gratitude is connected to self-talk; the words you say to yourself about on a regular basis.

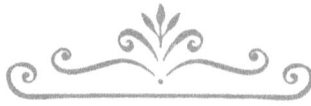

Lesson 17

Self-talk

Self-talk is something you do naturally throughout your waking hours. Positive self-talk is a powerful tool for increasing self-confidence and curbing negative emotions because it is supportive and affirming. Consider the following two inner statements and determine which is the more supportive: "I'm going to speak up in the meeting today. I have something important to contribute" or "I don't want to speak up in the meeting today. I'll look foolish if I say the wrong thing." Researchers find that it's not just about what you say to yourself, but the language you use to say it. Notice the labels you are using such as "the elderly" or "senior citizen." Think about the image and feelings those terms evoke for you.

A negative aspect of self-talk is the inner critic or the voice in the back of your mind that plays off your greatest fears. This inner voice comes from early experiences when a person witnesses, perceives, or experiences hurtful attitudes toward themselves or others. People unconsciously adopt and integrate these patterns of destructive thought, which then impact behavior and shape the direction of their lives. Negative self-talk can sabotage your plan to age optimally.

The inner critic's self-talk tends to fall into one of two categories: the "bad self" or the "weak self." The bad self is shame-based. Those who struggle with it may feel unlovable, flawed, inadequate, deserving of punishment, or incompetent. On the other hand, the weak self is fear and anxiety based. Those who struggle with it might feel dependent on others, unable to support themselves, submissive,

40

unable to express emotions for fear of something bad happening, vulnerable, mistrustful, deprived, or abandoned.

Awareness is the first step in recognizing and releasing the inner critic. Many people don't realize its presence. Notice the next time you are aware of feeling anxious, distracted, or numb. Identify the inner critic's voice and the situation that may have triggered it. Ask yourself the following questions, "What am I afraid of?" and "What would that mean?" Dig deeper and find your most vulnerable feelings about the situation.

One strategy for countering negative self-talk is to label the behavior rather than the person. Instead of saying to yourself "You were stupid to buy that computer" you could say "Buying a computer was not wise." The behavior was wrong not the person.

A second strategy is recommended by Byron Katie, a well-known American author and educator. In her book "*The Work*," Katie suggests using a set of four questions to challenge the inner critic. The four questions are:

1. Is it (the criticism) true?
2. Can you absolutely know it's true?
3. How do you react when you believe the inner critic?
4. Who would you be without the thought?

She then suggests turning the thought around. For example, if your thought was "she is mad at me." Then, turning it around might be "she isn't mad at me." At best the new thought will change your attitude and perhaps your behavior.

As you can see, a person's self-talk plays a major role in how he or she views aging. If you can no longer ski because of a torn ligament in your knee, you may tell yourself life is over or you may decide it's time to find a new sport - one that is not so hard on your knees.

PRACTICE

Use these strategies described above to evaluate what your inner critic saying to you. Is it helpful?

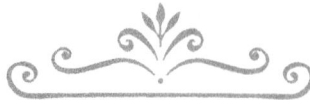

Lesson 18

Habits

A habit begins as a thought, a single thread. Every time the thought is repeated or reinforced, it grows stronger and becomes a stronger thread. Over time the thread becomes a thick cable, and as you may know a learned habit is often difficult to break.

Learned habits, instinctive behaviors and routines occur automatically without conscious intention or thought. These habits begin to form at birth and by age six most people have ingrained behaviors that remain throughout their lives.

Albert Einstein described insanity as doing the same thing over and over while expecting different results. So, in aging optimally you must identify outdated habits that are no longer useful and, in the process, you must examine underlying beliefs which maintain those habits.

One strategy is to examine habits of the mind employed by characteristically intelligent, successful people. According to the teachthought.com website as shown in the image below.[8]

Habits play a major role in your ability to age optimally. It is wise to review them and release those holding you back or keeping you stuck.

---

[8]   https://www.teachthought.com/pedagogy/what-are-the-habits-of-mind/

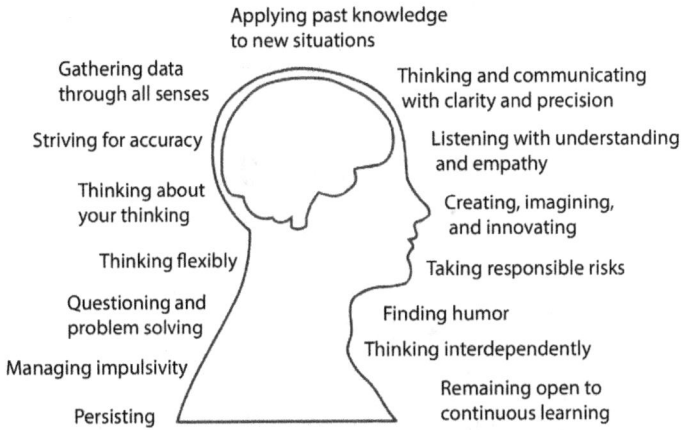

Applying past knowledge
to new situations

Gathering data
through all senses

Thinking and communicating
with clarity and precision

Striving for accuracy

Listening with understanding
and empathy

Thinking about
your thinking

Creating, imagining,
and innovating

Thinking flexibly

Taking responsible risks

Questioning and
problem solving

Finding humor

Thinking interdependently

Managing impulsivity

Remaining open to
continuous learning

Persisting

PRACTICE

Make a list of your habits: the behaviors you repeat regularly and tend to do unconsciously, such as biting your fingernails, rubbing your eyes, or exercising for 15 minutes every morning. Then ask yourself whether those habits are helpful or harmful.

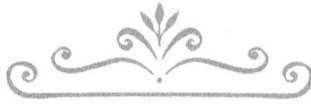

Lesson 19

Choice

Another factor to consider is choice. We have been given an incredible and irrevocable gift that provides us with the power to choose our life path but we must accept responsibility for the choices we make. How does choice influence a person's goal to age optimally? It seems clear that you can choose to live a healthy lifestyle: You can choose to see the cup half empty or half full; you can see an incident as good or bad; or you can choose to accept what others say as true or find what is true for you. The bottom line is that optimal aging is a choice and sometimes a tough choice given circumstance that inevitably arise.

An example would be DeShawn, a 60-year-old, wealthy retired man who was recently diagnosed with multiple sclerosis. His wife, DeLora, has dementia and their only child has leukemia. What might he choose? He could say to himself "woe is me" and give up or he could say "this is my new reality. These are my options and resources. How can I best approach this new normal?" He can also choose to talk with his wife and other family members and together make a plan for the future, which includes a larger support system, education, and a promise to each other to work as a team to do what is necessary.

PRACTICE

Think of a troublesome situation you are now facing and look at it through the lens of the cup being half full and half empty. What difference does it make?

44

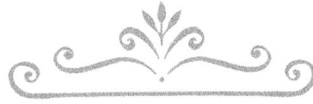

Lesson 20

Self-Care

Finally, aging optimally is a worthy goal but it can sometimes be challenging. Whether you are single or in a relationship, whether you and loved ones are healthy or experiencing health problems, whether things are going well or you are facing stressful issues, no matter the circumstances, self-care must be a top priority.

I suggest two options in your pursuit of self-care: a) develop a plan and b) set yourself up for success.

When you read online, you find many ideas for pampering yourself: such as taking a walk in the woods or enjoying a leisurely bubble bath. I found that many of those ideas didn't work for me. So, I took the time to explore what was important to me. My list included gardening, a daily glass of wine, doing things with family, being creative through writing and painting, having a meaningful purpose, being outdoors by the water as much as possible, and reading. Knowing that, I do four of those items for myself daily. I have flowers in the house and plants on the patio. I talk with my son and daughter daily. I have a glass of wine with dinner and every night I take a walk and read.

Your list may be different but for me setting myself up for success meant ensuring I look nice when I get up in the morning, doing what it takes to help me do my best easily and effectively, taking breaks. being kind to myself, forgiving my mistakes and unwise decisions, and asking myself daily "what more can I do?"

PRACTICE

Take the time to do this for yourself, now. Develop a self-care plan which includes setting yourself up for success. Such a plan could make a major difference in your life and your ability to age optimally.

Lesson 21

Retirement—Now What?

The lessons you have finished to this point are a sound foundation for aging optimally. However, difficult life circumstances can challenge the pursuit of that goal. Let's explore several of those potential circumstances briefly and identify which characteristics may be helpful and how. To begin with, let's use this example. Sixty-five-year-old Annie was forced with retirement from her job as a trainer. Money was not an issue and she thought writing a non-fiction book on motivational strategies and learning to play tennis would be fun. She had a wealth of experience to share and had always wanted to play tennis. However, after three months she was bored. She missed the challenge and structure of work, as well as the connection she shared with her co-workers and friends. Writing and tennis could not be the sole purpose for the rest of her life; she needed more stimulation.

Fortunately, Annie was willing to explore other possibilities. She read about optimal aging and conducted a personal housecleaning, re-examined her new normal, and revised her future plan. Her lifestyle was already healthy and she was very grateful for what she had; but she realized that she needed to redefine her purpose. After seriously considering her options, she found herself inspired to work with assault victims. So, she enrolled in a training for domestic violence advocates. Not only was this a valuable contribution to others but she also found that she could use her previous skills and include what she learned in her writing. This seemed liked a perfect addition to her purpose and she decided she would review the plan in six months.

PRACTICE

Consider carefully and honestly: Is retirement what you thought it would be or are you looking for something more?

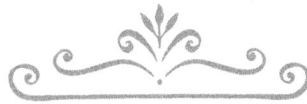

Lesson 22

Overcoming a Health Challenge

As people age, almost everyone has major or minor health challenges. Either way there are ways to handle them so that you can age optimally. For example, Sam is an older man who wants to live a long active life. Two years ago, he had sepsis, a life-threatening condition in which the body fights a severe infection that spreads through the bloodstream. As a result, doctors amputated his right leg and foot. He could no longer play golf and he had to sell his physical fitness/massage therapy business. He, now, has little confidence in driving or being socially active.

Sam had a very difficult time accepting his new restrictions and this newly imposed lifestyle. However, when he found a definition that said "to accept" meant acknowledging current reality without liking, wanting, or approving of it, he was able to move forward with his new normal which included many changes. He has limitations but this is who he is now. Nonetheless, he still has many options. He must accept that he can't change his situation, but he can control his actions and feelings. His life will never be the same, but there is still good to be had. He is responsible for his happiness no matter the circumstances. He must find new ways to earn a living and enjoy life.

Sam developed a plan to age optimally. He focused on perceptions and beliefs that are supportive. He accepted the facts that exist and use them to his advantage. He identified what he can do and what resources are available. He was grateful for what he has and keep a gratitude journal. Finally, he made healthy lifestyle choices as much as possible.

With this plan in mind, Sam was more able to accept his new normal and to adopt a more positive attitude; one that focused on aging optimally. When he experienced days of depression, he relied on his emotional resilience skills. He reminded himself that life wasn't always fair, that he must challenge his negative thoughts and rebuild his comfort level in social situations. After examining the alternatives, Sam chose to return to school and he enrolled in an online Psychology program. His new purpose was to work with clients experiencing physical disabilities such as his.

PRACTICE

Where could you apply this approach in your life right now?

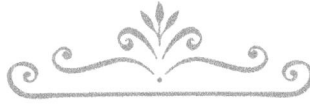

Lesson 23

A Loved One Faces a Terminal Illness

Aging optimally can be particularly challenging and heartbreaking when a loved one has a terminal illness. Julia is a 70-year-old woman whose husband, Dennis, has terminal cancer. She has taken over his care and the household duties. Most days she is compassionate and understands that he is ill, depressed, and in pain. Other days she feels overwhelmed, heartbroken, and frustrated. She misses their previous lifestyle and experiences deep discouragement about the future. He was her rock, her mainstay, and her best friend. She knows, though, that being discouraged and overwhelmed isn't helpful. So, let's look at Julia's attempt to manage her new normal.

Julia begins by focusing on doing her best and managing her emotions. With that in mind she formulates a goal by asking herself the following questions

- What do I want?
  JULIA: I want to accept Dennis's health condition without being demoralized by it.

- How will I know when I reach the goal? What do I want to happen?
  JULIA: Even though, I miss the way life was, my sadness and sense of loss won't overwhelm me. I will focus on what I can do rather than

what I can't do. I will continue to build good
memories with him and explore new interests.

- What will I hear, see, and feel as I achieve the goal?
  JULIA: I will hear myself talking about the positives,
  see myself being active and supportive, and feel
  good about life despite the circumstances.

- Why is my goal relevant?
  JULIA: I want to enjoy the rest of my life with Dennis
  and continue to be happy when he is no longer alive.

- What stops me from pursuing the goal wholeheartedly?
  JULIA: I tend to focus on what I no longer
  have. This means I get stuck in old habits and
  have trouble accepting this new normal.

- What personal resources can I use to achieve this goal?
  JULIA: I want to age optimally. My family
  is supportive, and I have good health.

- What additional resources do I need to achieve my goal?
  JULIA: I need to replace discouragement
  with a more optimistic mindset and I need
  to find additional purposes for life.

- How can the goal affect important people in my life and
  what risks are associated with achieving it?
  JULIA: My family is thrilled because I am
  seeking ways to move forward and they enjoy
  my company. Nonetheless, there is a risk that
  circumstances may cause me to lose focus.

- What daily actions must I take to achieve my goal, and
  what is the first step?
  JULIA: I need to monitor my self-talk, give myself
  some breaks, and adopt motivational strategies that
  help me remain strong. In addition, the FIRST STEP
  is to be thankful for and enjoy what I have now.

- Act, observe the results, and incorporate the feedback
  gained.

JULIA: I will try the options I know of, use what works, change what can be changed, and let go of what doesn't.

As a counselor had suggested, Julia asked her feelings what they needed. She thought about a time when she was particularly discouraged and allowed an image to come to mind. The image was of a heavy, black cloud. She drew the cloud on a piece of paper. Even though it seemed silly, she sat the picture on a chair across from her and asked the cloud what it needed and what she could do for it. The thought that came to mind was "I want to be there for Dennis with a positive attitude and have a plan for the future." She then placed the image of the black cloud in an imaginary balloon and released it into the sky.

Julia decided to better prepare herself now and in the future. She practiced emotional resilience so that she could manage the dark days and identified what she was motivated or inspired to pursue in the future such as volunteering, learning something new, or traveling. Even though she wasn't sure what the future held she was willing to be creative.

PRACTICE

Think about a time when you were discouraged. What image comes to mind? Draw the image on a piece of paper and ask the image what it needs from you or what its message is for you. The image just might reveal an important lesson.

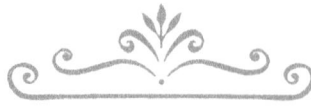

Lesson 24

Balancing Goals—Yours and Your Partner's

Sometimes you and your partner are on different paths: heading in different directions. As my daughter once said "It's like you are 70 going on 60 and Dad is 70 going on 80." So, let's look at how a person can age optimally given that situation. Pritha handled it this way. She and Ragesh have been married for 50 years. Since retiring, Ragesh had found no hobbies, has no interest in learning anything new, and refuses to travel or volunteer. While he is healthy physically, he is also a very private man. His perceived ailments and his hearing loss provide additional excuses for him not doing many things.

Pritha read about aging optimally and wants to pursue this lifestyle. She has a lot of energy, wants to do things, but chooses not to if Ragesh doesn't want to. She can only leave for short periods of time because he broods and makes questionable decisions. It is difficult for her to move forward with her goals and dreams given this situation. She wants to be there for him, but she also wants her own life.

Pritha assessed her new normal. She realized several facts: Ragesh probably won't change, she wants to spend the rest of her life with him, she must take on more of the responsibilities, to survive she must honor herself more, and although she is interested in aging optimally, he is not.

Based on that assessment Pritha developed a plan. She decided to balance pursing her goals, friends, and dreams as much as possible while doing things with Ragesh he could and would do. She managed the household tasks, while allowing Ragesh to do what he can. She learned mindfulness and meditation skills. She adopted an optimistic attitude and a resourceful mind set. The final parts of Pritha's plan were to change her beliefs and self-talk about what she could and couldn't do and to release long held habits - ones in which they did things together and had similar interests and goals. Her mantra became "I think I can, I think I can!!" "I know I can!!"

PRACTICE

Do you and your partner have the same goals? If not, take the time to find ways to honor both of your needs as you age optimally. Be creative!

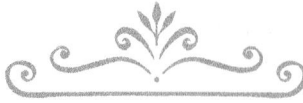

Lesson 25

Transitions Due to Mental Health Issues

Another major challenge for someone wishing to age optimally is a mental health issue of a loved one. So, let's take a look at how Ebony manages her situation. Issac has dementia and gets confused easily. They considered selling their condo and moving to a retirement community which included assisted living and memory care facilities if and when necessary and even visited several communities. However, they did not like what they saw and the cost was enormous. So, they decided to remain where they were presently. This means that Ebony must take on greater responsibility and a greater role in managing their lives. In the future, it may mean require outside help.

Because she wants to age optimally, Ebony redefined her new normal. She accepted that Issacs's condition was part of her life now and that she must take charge to a greater degree. Her plan included to set limits, to forgive herself for getting frustrated, and to remember that he needs extra help. Her goals include learning more about dementia and managing the behaviors involved, responding to his questions and interruptions patiently, giving him limited choices, and not reasoning with him. Ebony also knows she must take care of herself or she won't be available to carry out her plan.

PRACTICE

If your loved one has either physical or mental health issues, you must take care of yourself first or you won't be available to support them. Take the time now to develop a care plan for yourself; then when needed you will be better able to help your loved one.

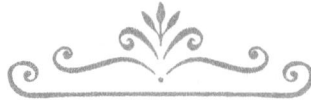

Lesson 26

Adapting to a New Role

Sometimes, even oftentimes, life situations change and to age optimally you must change habits, behaviors, and beliefs. Take a look at Debbie's situation. Cheng always managed the family finances and he did an excellent job. Because of recent health issues, he was forced to retire. He had worked his entire life; so, it scared him when he was no longer bringing in a paycheck. Based on his fear, he sold a large amount of stock and then vehemently denied that he did: even though there was evidence to the contrary.

Once Debbie realized this, she revised her new normal and adapted her purpose to include learning about finances and taking over their financial management. She revised her perceptions and beliefs regarding her abilities to do those tasks and changed her habit of letting him take charge. Two other considerations for Debbie were that she was mourning the loss of the person she knew and she needed to appreciate herself for the tasks she was accomplishing.

One new habit Debbie adopted was to meditate three times a day: on waking, at noon, and before bedtime. Her meditation practice is short - three to five minutes each session. She found this provided a calming effect, quieted her worries, and allowed her to have a better night's sleep.

PRACTICE

For the next week, embrace Debbie's example. Meditate three times a day for three to five minutes and at the end of the week write down the benefits you have noticed. If meditation doesn't work for you, figure out why not. Are your thoughts overwhelming? Are you unable to stay focused? If so, visit Lesson 14.

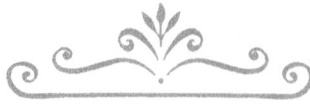

Apathy with Life

Sometimes life throws us curves that we are not able to rise above. Consequently, a low-level depression and apathy seeps in. At this time a good friend can play a major role. For example, at age 60, Mike was fired from his long-held position as an accountant for a local tech company because his drinking had gotten worse. Mike is divorced, he had no plans or no real reason for living. He is worried about money, depressed and furious with himself for getting fired.

Mike was immobilized and couldn't move forward, so his best friend, Jose, who knew about aging optimally, stepped in. He assessed Mike's new normal and identified that while Mike did not have a job currently, he was financially well-off. Mike was fired for drinking, but his drinking was a recent problem due to his unhappiness with his work. He had skills and years of experience. He was not open to aging optimally, but Jose cared enough about his friend to take the initiative.

After the assessment, he developed a plan to motivate Mike without his realizing it. The plan had five parts. The first part was to encourage Mike to get help for the drinking and he offered to attend A-A meetings with him. The second part was to take Mike to meet with a mutual friend who was a career counselor to explore his options. He also took Mike to play golf and they joined a club. Finally, he created a list of projects to help him build self-confidence and asked Mike's out of town family members to support him.

It took, a couple of months but Mike did get a new job and he was relatively happy even though he was still not interested in the goal of aging optimal.

PRACTICE

Do you know of someone who is apathetic or do you feel apathetic at times? This type of plan may allow you to step in; to get him, her, or even you going again.

Lesson 28

Money Worries

A major concern for many older adults is having enough money. Take Darnell's story for example. At age 60, Darnell worries that he will not have enough money to live comfortably after he retires or if he gets laid off. He thinks about his bills and his savings, as well as how long he and his wife might live and their hopes and dreams. He doesn't see how they can survive financially if they remain on their current path.

Darnell read Byron Katie's inquiry method and her set of four questions.[9] He decided to use them to challenge his worry.

When Darnell asked himself the following questions, these were his responses

1. What thoughts and beliefs are present?
   DARNELL: I keep thinking I won't have enough money to retire and still enjoy life. I might lose my job or be forced to get a second job to pay the bills. I don't believe I have the skills or energy to get another job.
2. What feelings are present?
   DARNELL: I am constantly worried that I won't be able to provide for my family.
3. What body sensations are here now?
   DARNELL: I feel heaviness in my chest, tension in my shoulders, and my head aches constantly.

---

[9] https://www.habitsforwellbeing.com/inquiry-4-questions-that-can-change-your-life-from-byron-katie/

4. What do I need to pay attention to right now?
    DARNELL: I really need to pay more attention
    to my finances and expenses to determine
    whether I need to be concerned.
5. When he asked himself Byron Katie's original four
    questions, his answers were as follows
6. Is it true that you don't have enough money to live after
    retirement?
    DARNELL: Maybe
7. Can you know that it is absolutely true?
    DARNELL: No, not really.
8. How do you react when you believe you don't have
    enough money?
    DARNELL: I get anxious and self-critical; I have
    migraine headaches and my IBS acts up.
9. Who would you be without that thought?
    DARNELL: I would be confident that I
    am financially stable and could relax.

Realizing this encouraged Darnell to meet with a financial planner to get a sense of his financial picture. After that meeting, he and his wife were motivated to complete a plan. The plan included saving a certain amount of money each month. They also willingly looked at their spending habits and made the choice to let go of habits that were not benefitting them. This was a great first step for them as they aged optimally.

Do you have money worries? Do you understand what your financial future will be? If not decide today to investigate it today. Knowing what the future holds is always less scary than guessing.

PRACTICE

One way to proceed is to begin by writing down a list of your assets including future Social Security benefits. Then make a list of your expenses and assess whether or not your expenses are greater than your earnings. Finally, identify where to cut back and what you need to save. Once you are armed with this information, you can meet with a financial planner who will help you develop a financial plan. So, take advantage of this outside help because it will remove worries and set you on a good financial path.

Lesson 29

Your Partner Has a Chronic Illness

Sometimes, your loved one has a progressive, long-term illness as Jade does. Jade is a 60-year-old female, who was recently diagnosed with early stage ALS or amyotrophic lateral sclerosis. ALS is the progressive neurodegenerative disease that affects nerve cells in the brain and the spinal cord. She and her partner are interested in aging optimally so they take a very proactive approach in managing their lives and their emotions. A team of neurologists are treating her disease.

After reading many articles online, they feel that the lifestyle aspects of optimal aging are a sound foundation for moving forward. They assessed their new normal and then drafted a plan to age optimally within that new normal. They wanted to make the best of it now while preparing for the future.

Their plan included taking trips, while she is still able, learning French because they want to visit Paris, Nice, and Monaco, saving money for the future, and volunteering at an animal shelter. They continued to read about new ways to manage her health issues, to eat nutritiously, and to exercise regularly. Finally, they chose to be grateful for what they had every day and they practiced mindfulness. That was the easy part. They both needed to learn and practice emotional resilience. Jade's disease was chronic and fatal; so, they needed to find ways to regularly manage their emotions. They chose to experiment with several ideas. They kept a journal, together, focused on what they did have and the good parts of the day, remained optimistic, and sought additional   resources. Even so, there were days of discouragement and they needed to rely on the support of friends.

PRACTICE

If your loved one or friend has a chronic illness, you will want to make a similar plan to best use the time you have together and be prepared for the future. A question to consider is "When he or she is gone, will we have done what we wanted?

Unexpected Changes

Life is full of change. Some of those changes are positive and others negative. As a way of aging optimally, you will want to find a way to view the positive aspect of negative changes such as Leon did. He was furious because his wife of 40 years, Latoya, left him recently for a man she met on the Internet. This was unexpected. When he thought about the situation, he felt pressure in his head, told himself repeatedly that this wasn't fair and that he didn't deserve it. Yet, for the sake of his children and his own well-being he really didn't want to be vindictive and hateful toward her. They had experienced many good years together.

Leon knew about the new behavior generator in which a person does the following:

1. **Identifies a positive behavior outcome.** For example, remaining calm in aggravating situations.
2. **States the new behavior in positive terms.** The goal would be to remain calm rather than to not get aggravated.
3. **Creates an imaginary movie depicting a picture of the behavior he or she wishes to possess.** This can be of another person or a time when the behavior effectively. The role model chosen can be someone personally known, a celebrity, a TV character or even an animal. Change the vision of the movie until it is exactly how it should be: what is thought, felt, and done.

4. **Checks how the body feels while doing the behavior.**
    Consider what posture is like when talking to someone
    calmly and patiently.
5. **Tries it out.** In order to test this new behavior in a real-life
    situation, be thoroughly convinced that the new behavior
    has been learned.

So, with that in mind, Leon decided he wanted to respond
as graciously and respectfully as George Herbert Walker Bush had
responded when he was not re-elected president. Leon practiced
being respectful and gracious in the face of irritating situations. He
pictured (made a movie in his mind) seeing Latoya as they went
through the divorce settlement and responding with grace - telling
her how he was building a new life for himself and how appreciative
he was for their time together. After practicing numerous times,
Leon was able to think about the divorce as a positive event and a
new beginning. He did see his ex-wife in social settings and was able
to be cordial with her.

Granted, there were times when he was sad, but he decided not
to dwell on the past and to be grateful for where he was presently. He
actively looked for a new special person in his life and found other
activities where he might meet people with similar interests and get
reconnected with life.

PRACTICE

We all experience changes. Some are startling and others are life
altering such as Leon's. Have you experienced any stunning life
changes? How did you deal with them? What worked for you? What
didn't work and why? What works for you currently?

Final Thoughts

In this booklet you have been provided with a series of lessons for getting ready to age optimally. For a much more in-depth discussion of aging optimally look for the booklet, Ten Guidelines for Aging Optimally that will be coming soon. Remember this:

"Aging is an opportunity not a disease" (author unknown)

JANICE WALTON, PHD

Thank You

Thank you for taking the time to read this book. I hope you found it valuable. Here are some final take-aways you might find useful for further advancement.

- For more material and resources like this, please check my website here: **www.tlcorner.com**

- I am always adding material to the site, so if you don't find what you need, do make sure to check back or send me a note.

- To be kept informed of future publications, you can **join my mailing list**.

Finally, if you found this book valuable, would you **please leave a review on Amazon or Goodreads?**

My commitment is to add as much value as possible for you to achieve your life goals. Your interest in my materials is hugely appreciated, and I hope you will consider these options and future publications.

Best wishes,
Janice Walton, PhD

www.ingramcontent.com/pod-product-compliance
Lightning Source LLC
Chambersburg PA
CBHW071931020426
42331CB00010B/2812